Your Plant-Based Diet Breakfast

An Introduction to Plant-Based Breakfast Recipes to Boost Your Day and Manage Your Weight

Dave Ingram

Table of contents

Cranberry Apple Cider Pie

Cook time: 60 minutes

Servings: 6-8

Ingredients:

1/2 cup tap water 2 cups cranberries

2 orange zest and juice 1/2 cup maple syrup 1/3 cup sugar

4 cups apples, peeled and sliced 3/4 teaspoon cinnamon

1/2 teaspoon pumpkin pie spice

2 cups + 1 1/2 tablespoons all-purpose flour 1 1/4 teaspoon salt

2 2/3 tablespoons vegan butter 6 tablespoons of ice water

Instructions:

1.   Preheat the oven to 400F. Mix tap water, maple syrup, and cranberries in a pan. Boil and stir for 10 minutes. Remove and let cool.

5

2.   Peel and slice apples into pieces. Mix with 1/3 cup sugar, 1/4 teaspoon salt, 1/2 teaspoon cinnamon, 1/4 tsp pumpkin pie spice, and 1 1/2 tablespoons flour.

3.   Whisk the remaining flour, salt, cinnamon, and pumpkin pie spice in a bowl. Add butter and mix until crumbly. Add ice water and mix well until the dough forms. Shape the dough into 2 balls, one bigger than the other ones.

4.   Roll the more giant ball into the crust and place it on a pie pan. Mix cranberry sauce and apple filling and add to the pan with the dough.

5.   Roll out the other dough ball. Press down the edges and sprinkle with sugar and cinnamon.

6.   Bake for 45 minutes. Let cool completely.

7.   Serve and enjoy.

Vegan Chocolate Avocado Pudding

Cook Time: 20 minutes

Servings: 6

Ingredients:

1 large banana

1 1/2 avocados

1/4 cup any sweetener 1/2 cup cacao powder

1/4 cup almond milk, unsweetened mixed berries for topping

Instructions:

1.   Add all ingredients to a blender and blend until thoroughly combined and smooth.

2. Transfer to a bowl, add toppings and serve.

Rosemary Fig Scones

Cook Time: 40 minutes

Servings: 8

Ingredients:

1/4 cup coconut sugar 2 cups brown rice flour

1/2 cup coconut oil, cold

1 tbsp baking powder 1 cup milk

3 tablespoons rosemary, chopped 1 tablespoon lemon zest

1/2 cup dry figs, chopped 1/4 teaspoon salt

Instructions:

1.   Preheat the oven to 350F.

2.   Mix rosemary, lemon zest, and milk in a bowl and set aside.

3.   Mix coconut sugar, brown rice flour, baking powder, coconut oil, and salt in a bowl. Add coconut oil

into the flour mixture and stir to combine. Add dried figs into it.

4.   Mix dry and wet ingredients and make the dough. Roll out the dough into a circle about 1 1/2" thick. Cut the dough into 8 pieces.

5.   Bake for 18 minutes.

6. Serve and enjoy.

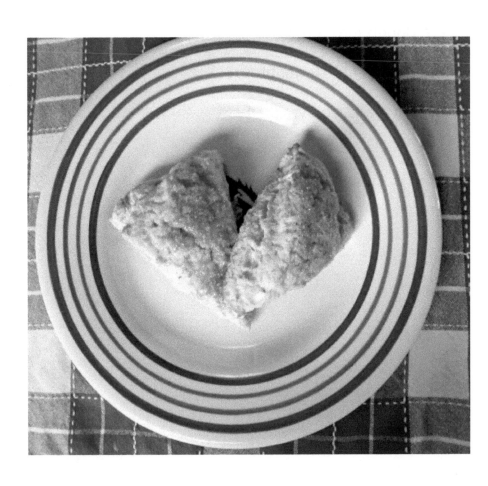

Carrot Cake Waffles

Cook Time: 15 minutes

Servings: 4

Ingredients:

1   cup flour, gluten-free

2   tbsp coconut sugar 1/2 tsp cinnamon

1 teaspoon baking powder

1 1/2 tablespoons ground flax seeds 3/4 cup almond milk

1 tsp apple vinegar 1/2 cup carrots, grated

2   1/2 tablespoons warm water 1/4 cup pineapple, crushed

2 tablespoon coconut flakes 1 pinch ground ginger

1 pinch salt

Instructions:

1.   Preheat waffle iron. Stir almond milk and vinegar. Add warm water to the flax seeds to make the flax egg.

2. Mix the dry ingredients and combine well. Add almond milk mixture, coconut, and crushed pineapple to it and mix.

3. Add the grated carrots and flax egg. Cook until crispy and golden.

4. Serve and enjoy.

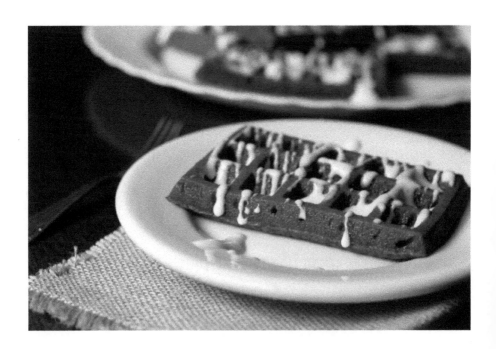

High Protein Dessert Pizza with Raspberry Sauce

Cook Time: 30 minutes

Servings: 4

Ingredients:

½ glass chickpea flour 1/2 glass cacao powder

1 packet Plant Fusion Lean Chocolate Brownie Flavor 3 tablespoons maple syrup

2 tablespoons coconut oil 1/2 teaspoon vanilla extract 1 cup coconut cream

1 lemon, zested

12 oz. raspberries

1 tablespoon lemon juice

Instructions:

1.   Preheat the oven to 350F.

2.   Mix Plant Fusion Lean, chickpea flour, and cacao powder in a bowl. Mix 2 tablespoons of maple syrup and

coconut oil. Add to the dry ingredients and mix until smooth.

3.   Roll out the dough into a circle. Place onto parchment paper. Bake for 14 minutes and let cool.

4.   Mix raspberries, lemon zest, and juice in a pot. Bring to a boil and cook until jam-like consistency forms and let cool.

5.   Beat coconut milk in a bowl on high for 2 minutes. Add vanilla extract and maple syrup and beat until well mixed.

6.   Cut the pizza crust into 8 pieces, top with raspberries, raspberry jam, coconut cream, and serve.

High Protein, Raw Vegan Carrot Cake

Cook time: 5 minutes

Servings: 4

Ingredients:

1/2 cup dried coconut 2 carrots

1/2 cup ground almonds 2 tablespoons orange zest 2 tablespoons orange juice 1 teaspoon cinnamon

2 teaspoon stevia

1/4 tsp nutmeg 1/2 cup pecans

3 tablespoon vanilla protein powder 2 tablespoons lemon juice

2 cups soaked cashews

2 tablespoon maple syrup 2 tablespoon coconut oil Water

Instructions:

1.   Blend the first 10 ingredients in a blender until smooth. Add the blended mix to a cake pan. Bake for about 45-50 minutes.

2.   Blend the remaining ingredients until smooth.

3.   Add frosting over the cake and serve.

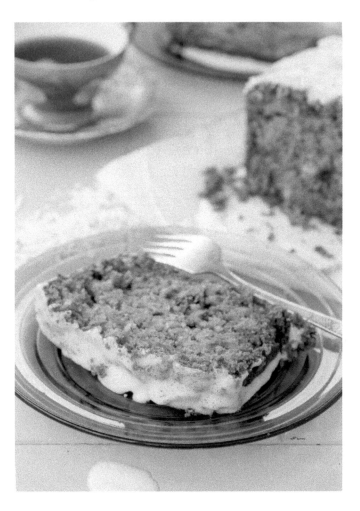

Glory Muffins

Total time: 30 minutes

Ingredients

1¾ cups flour

½ teaspoon baking powder

½ cup sugar

2 teaspoons cinnamon

½ teaspoon ground ginger 3 flax eggs

1 cup plant-based milk

½ cup maple syrup

1 teaspoon vanilla extract 1 apple, shredded

2 carrots, shredded

1 teaspoon baking soda

⅓ cup walnuts, chopped

½ teaspoon salt

Directions

1.   Preheat the oven to 180°.

2.   Mix flaxseed with water in a bowl and leave for 10 minutes.

3.   In a bowl, mix flour, sugar, ginger, cinnamon, baking soda, salt, and baking powder.

4.   Stir in vanilla, maple syrup, and milk along with flaxseed mix.

5.   Mix well to make a batter, then fold in apple, nuts, and carrots.

6.   Line a muffin tin with 6 muffin cups and divide the carrot batter evenly between them.

7.   Bake for 20 minutes, then serve.

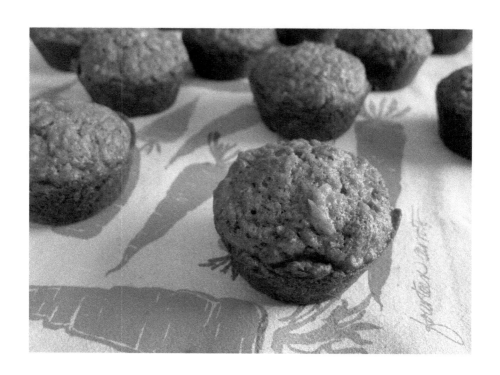

Amazing Almond & Banana Granola

Total time: 75 minutes

Ingredients:

2 peeled and chopped ripe bananas 8 cups of rolled oats

1 teaspoon of salt

2 cups of freshly pitted and chopped dates 1 cup of slivered and toasted almonds

1 teaspoon of almond extract

Directions

1.   Preheat the oven to 275o F.

2.   Line two 13 x 18-inch baking sheets with parchment paper.

3.   In a medium saucepan, add 1 cup of water and the dates, and bring to a boil. Cook for 15 minutes. The dates will be soft and pulpy. Keep on adding water to the saucepan so that the dates do not stick to the pan.

4.   After removing the dates from the heat, allow them to cool before you blend them with salt, almond extract, and bananas.

5.   You will have a smooth and creamy puree.

6.   Add this mixture to the oats, and give it a thorough mix.

7.   Divide the mixture into equal halves and spread over the baking sheets.

8.   Bake for about 30-40 minutes, stirring every 10 minutes or so.

9.   The granola will be ready when crispy.

10.   After removing the baking sheets from the oven, allow them to cool. Then, add the slivered almonds.

High Protein Rice Crispie Treats

Cook Time: 10 minutes

Servings: 8 treats

Ingredients:

1/4 cup vanilla plant-based protein powder 2 cups crisp rice cereal

3 tablespoons brown rice syrup 3 tablespoons creamy nut butter

Instructions:

1.   Grease an 8 cup muffin tin. Mix protein powder and cereal in a bowl.

2.   Heat a pan over medium heat. Cook the syrup and nut butter until mixtures start bubbling. Cook for 30 seconds longer.

3.   Add over cereal mixture and stir well. Add to the prepared muffin cups.

4.   Cool completely, remove and serve.

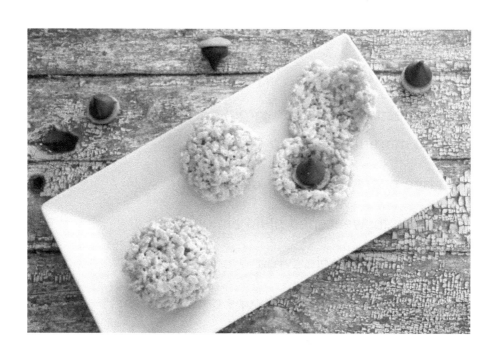

Maple Pear Oatmeal

Preparation time: 8 minutes

Cook time: 30 minutes

Serves 6

Ingredients:

2 tablespoons organic virgin coconut oil, melted, plus a little more for greasing the pan

3 ripe pears, cored and diced

2 cups unsweetened plain almond milk

¼ cup pure maple syrup

1 tbsp vanilla extract 2 cups oats

¾ cup chopped pecans

½ cup raisins

1 teaspoon ground cinnamon

½ teaspoon ground ginger

¼ teaspoon ground nutmeg

¼ teaspoon sea salt

Directions:

1. Turn on the oven. Distribute the pears in the bottom of the pan.

2. Wisk almond milk, maple syrup, vanilla, and melted oil.

3. Mix together the oats, pecans, raisins, cinnamon, ginger, nutmeg, and salt. Add the almond milk mixture and stir well. Spread evenly over the pears.

4. Bake until the center is set.

Morning Glory Breakfast Cookies

Preparation time: 8 minutes

Cook time: 20 minutes

Makes 12 large cookies

Ingredients:

1   cups gluten-free rolled oats 1 cup almond flour

¼ cup chia seeds

1 teaspoon baking soda

½ teaspoon ground cinnamon

½ teaspoon sea salt

1 cup mashed ripe banana

½ cup cashew butter

¼ cup coconut oil 1 tsp vanilla extract

¾ cup pitted dates, chopped

½ cup unsweetened shredded coconut

½ cup raw cashews, chopped

Directions:

1.   Heat the oven to 180ºC. Line 2 baking sheets with parchment paper.

2.   Stir the oats, almond flour or meal, chia seeds, baking soda, cinnamon, and salt. In another bowl, combine the banana, cashew butter, oil, and vanilla.

3.   Pour the banana mixture into the well and stir until thoroughly combined. Fold in the dates, coconut, and cashews.

4.   Using a $1/3$-cup measuring cup, drop small mounds of the dough onto the baking sheets, leaving a little space between each mound. There should be 12 large cookies. Gently press on the tops to flatten slightly.

5.   Bake for 20 minutes, or until the tops are golden brown.

Irish-Style Oatmeal

Preparation time: 5 minutes

Cook time: 30 minutes

Serves 4

Ingredients:

4 cups water

¼ teaspoon sea salt

1 cup gluten-free steel-cut oats 1 tablespoon pure maple syrup 1 tablespoon almond butter Suggested Toppings:

1 ripe banana, sliced

½ cup sliced almonds Dash of ground cinnamon

Directions:

1.   Add the oats to the boiling water and stir well. Cook 30 to 40 minutes. The oats will be chewy, but they should not have any crunch.

2. Mix the maple syrup and almond butter, then spoon the oatmeal into 4 bowls. If using any suggested toppings, add them now.

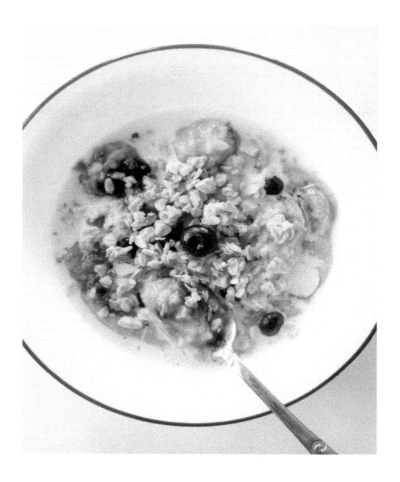

Coconut-Pecan Granola

Preparation time: 5 minutes

Cook time: 25 minutes

Serves 8

Ingredients:

2 cups gluten-free rolled oats

2 cup coconut 1 cup pecans, roughly chopped

1/3 cup almond meal

½ cup pure maple syrup

¼ cup organic virgin coconut oil, melted 2 teaspoons pure vanilla extract

¼ teaspoon ground cinnamon

¼ teaspoon sea salt

Directions:

1.   Heat the oven to 180ºC.

2.   Mix together the oats, coconut, pecans, and almond meal.

3.   Stir together the maple syrup, oil, vanilla, cinnamon, and salt. Pour the maple mixture over the oats mixture and stir well to coat everything.

4.   Bake for 10 minutes, then stir, spread again in an even layer, and bake for until toasted.

5.   Let cool completely. Store at room temperature.

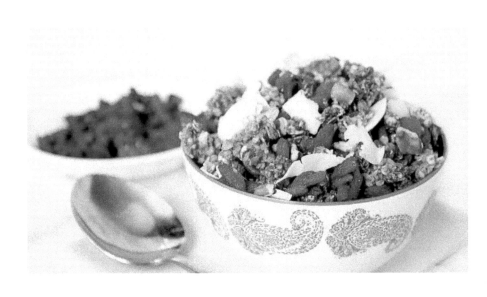

Chocolate Peanut Butter Shake

Preparation Time: 5 minutes

Cooking Time: 5 minutes

Servings: 2 servings

Ingredients:

2 bananas

3 Tablespoons peanut butter 1 cup almond milk

3 Tablespoons cacao powder

Directions:

1. Combine ingredients in a blender until smooth.

Nutrition:

Calories: 149 Fat: 1.1g Carbs: 1.5g Protein: 7.9g

Berries and Banana Smoothie Bowl

Preparation Time: 5 minutes

Cooking Time: 0 minutes

Servings: 4

Ingredients:

For the Smoothie:

4 cups frozen mixed berries

4 small frozen bananas, sliced

4 scoops of vanilla Protein: powder

12 tablespoons almond milk, unsweetened

For the Toppings:

4 tablespoons chia seeds

4 tablespoons shredded coconut, unsweetened

Directions:

4 tablespoons hemp seeds

½ cup Granola

Fresh strawberries, sliced, as needed

1.   Add mixed berries into a food processor and banana and then pulse at low speed for 1 to 2 minutes until broken.

2.   Add remaining ingredients for the smoothie and then pulse again for 1 minute at low speed until creamy, scraping the container's sides frequently.

3.   Distribute the smoothie among four bowls, then top with chia seeds, coconut, hemp seeds, granola, and strawberries and serve.

Nutrition:

Calories: 214 Fat: 2.5g Carbs: 47.5g Protein: 2.8g

Pomegranate Overnight Oats

Total time: 10 minutes

Ingredients

½ cup rolled oats

½ cup almond milk

½ cup pomegranate seeds

1 tablespoon ground flax seeds 1 tablespoon cocoa nibs

To Garnish:

¼ cup pomegranate seeds 2 teaspoon coconut shreds

Directions

1.   In a sealable container, add everything and mix well.

2.   Seal the container and refrigerate overnight.

3.   Serve with coconut shreds and pomegranate seeds on top.

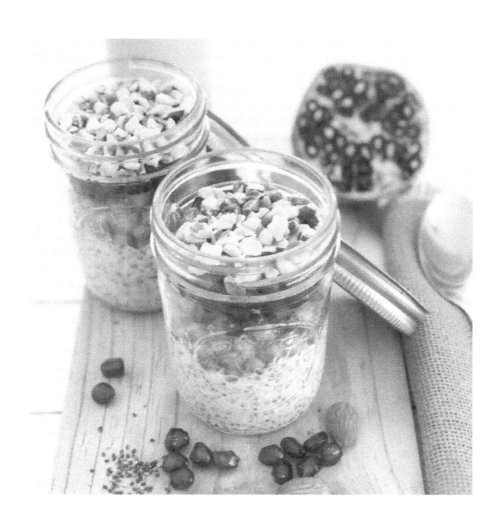

Almond Chia Pudding

Total time: 10 minutes

Ingredients

3 tablespoons almond butter 2 tablespoons maple syrup
1 cup almond milk

¼ cup plus 1 tablespoon chia seeds

Directions

1.   In a sealable container, add everything and mix well.

2.   Seal the container and refrigerate overnight.

3.   Serve with a splash of almond milk.

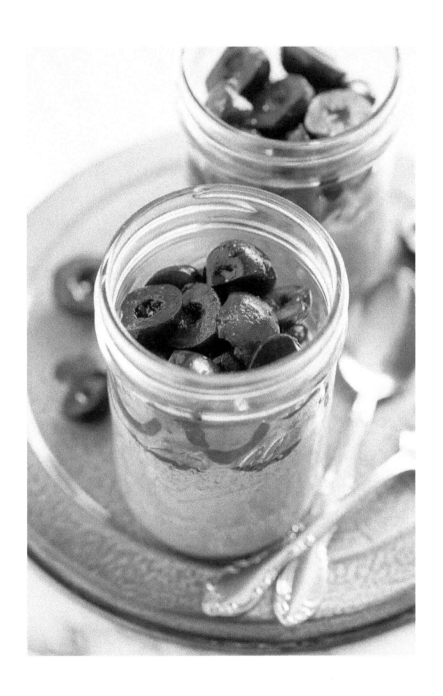

Toast with Tomato

Preparation time: 10 minutes

Cook time: 0 minutes

Makes 2 slices

Ingredients:

2 large slices of toast

1 garlic clove, halved 1 Roma tomato, halved Salt, to taste

Nutritional yeast (optional)

Directions:

1.   Rub each slice of toast with a garlic clove half and half a Roma tomato. Sprinkle with salt and, if desired, nutritional yeast.

Easy Avocado Toast

Preparation time: 10 minutes

Cook time: 0 minutes

Makes 2 slices

Ingredients:

1 ripe avocado, halved, pitted, and sliced 2 large slices of toast

Salt, to taste (optional)

Directions:

1.   Spread the avocado onto the toast. Sprinkle with salt, if desired.

Sunrise Smoothie

Preparation Time: 5 minutes

Cooking Time: 0 minutes

Servings: 4

Ingredients:

4 tablespoons chia seed 2 frozen banana

2 lemon, peeled

2 cups diced carrots 4 clementines, peeled

4 cups frozen strawberries, unsweetened 12 tablespoons pomegranate tendrils

2 cup almond milk, unsweetened

Directions:

1.   Put the ingredients in a blender and then pulse for 1 to 2 minutes until blended, scraping the sides of the container frequently.

2.   Distribute the smoothie among glasses and then serve.

Nutrition: 274 Cal 5.4 g Fat 0.5 g Saturated Fat 57.3 g Carbohydrates 13.3 g Fiber 33.8 g Sugars 0.5 g Protein

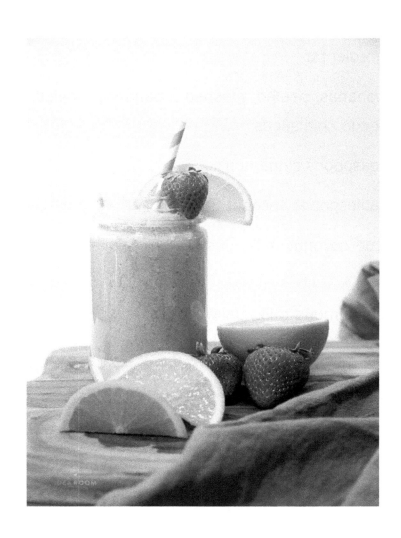

Banana Cream Pie and Chia Pudding

Preparation Time: 1 hour and 10 minutes

Cooking Time: 0 minutes

Servings: 4

Ingredients:

2 bananas, peeled, mashed 2 bananas, peeled, chopped

1/2 cup chia seeds

2 teaspoons cinnamon

4 tablespoons coconut flakes

1 cup coconut milk, unsweetened 2 tablespoons maple syrup

1 cup almond milk, unsweetened

Directions:

1.   Take a large bowl, add chia seeds and mashed bananas, add maple syrup and cinnamon, pour in almond and coconut milk, and whisk until well combined.

2.   Place the bowl in the refrigerator for a minimum of 1 hour until firm.

3.   When ready to eat, distribute pudding evenly among 4 bowls, top with chopped banana, and sprinkle with coconut flakes and then serve.

Nutrition:

Calories: 350 Fat: 17g Carbs: 37g Sugars: 19g Protein: 5g

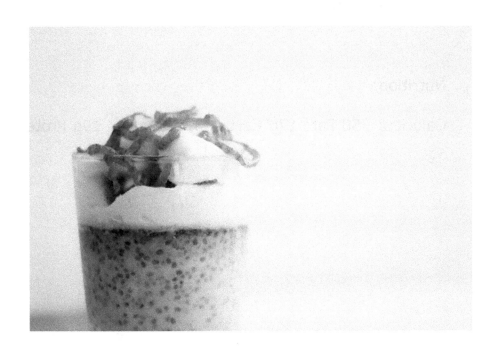

Brown Rice Breakfast Pudding

Preparation Time: 5 minutes

Cooking Time: 15 minutes

Servings: 4

Ingredients:

1 tart apple, cored, chopped

1 cup Medjool dates, pitted, chopped 3 cups cooked brown rice

1/8 teaspoon salt

¼ teaspoon ground cloves 1 cinnamon stick

¼ cup raisins

¼ cup slivered almonds, toasted

2 cups almond milk, unsweetened

Directions:

1.   Take a medium saucepan, place it over medium-low heat, add rice, dates, cloves, and cinnamon, pour in

milk, stir until mixed and cook for 12 minutes until thickened.

2.   Then remove and discard cinnamon stick, add apple and raisins and then stir in salt.

3.   Remove pan from heat, distribute pudding among four bowls, and top with almonds.

4.   Serve straight away.

Nutrition:

Calories: 391 Fat: 4.8g Carbs: 81.1g Sugars: 24.8g Protein: 6g

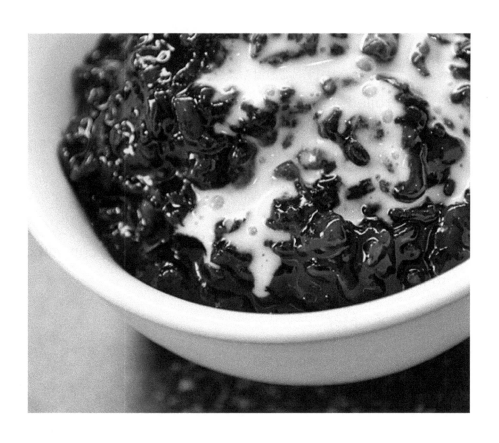

Oats with Chia

Preparation Time: 6 hours and 10 minutes

Cooking Time: 0 minutes

Servings: 4

Ingredients:

3 cups rolled oats

4 tablespoons chia seeds and more for topping 4 tablespoons maple syrup

1 teaspoon cinnamon

1 teaspoon vanilla extract, unsweetened 1 cup almond milk, unsweetened

2 cups of water

1 cup sliced strawberries

Directions:

1. Take an enormous container, add oats and chia seeds in it, add cinnamon, vanilla extract, and maple

syrup, then pour in water and almond milk and stir until mixed.

2.   Place the bowl in the refrigerator for a minimum of 6 hours.

3.   When ready to eat, distribute oats and chia mixture evenly among 4 bowls, top with some chia seeds and sliced strawberries, and then serve.

Nutrition:

Calories: 351.8 Fat: 7.4g Carbs: 62.4g Sugars: 14.6g Protein: 8.8g

Tempeh Maple Breakfast Sausage

Preparation time: 15 minutes

Cook time: 30 minutes

Makes 8 to 12 patties

Ingredients:

1 (8-ounce / 227-g) package tempeh, lightly steamed if desired, cubed 2 tablespoons maple syrup

2 tbsp flour 1 tbsp extra-virgin olive oil

1 tablespoon red miso 1 teaspoon dried sage

½ teaspoon dried rosemary

¼ teaspoon black pepper

⅛ teaspoon crushed red pepper

Directions:

1.   Heat the oven to 205°. Line a baking sheet with parchment paper.

2.   Place the tempeh in the bowl of a food processor. Add the maple syrup, flour, oil, miso, sage, rosemary,

black pepper, and crushed red pepper and pulse to combine.

3.   Transfer to a medium bowl and, using wet hands, form the mixture into 8 burger-size patties or 12 slider-sized ones.

4.   Bake for 30 minutes (for burger-size patties) or 20 minutes (for slider-sized patties), flipping halfway through. Serve.

Mint Chocolate Green Protein Smoothie

Preparation Time: 5 minutes

Cooking Time: 10 minutes

Servings: 1 serving

Ingredients:

1 scoop chocolate powder 1 tablespoon flaxseed

1 banana

1 mint leaf

3/4 cup almond milk

3 tablespoons dark chocolate (chopped)

Directions:

1.   Blend the ingredients without the dark chocolate.

2.   Garnish dark chocolate when ready.

Nutrition:

Calories: 300 Fat: 19.1g Carbs: 21.5g Protein: 27.9g

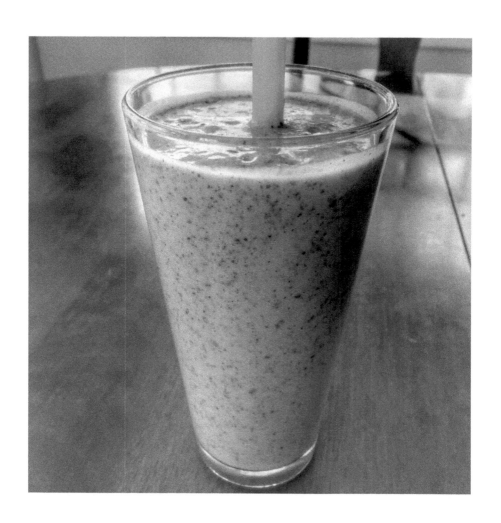

Banana Walnut Crunch Loaf

Preparation time: 5 minutes

Cook time: 1 hour

Makes 1 loaf

Ingredients:

4 ripe bananas

¼ cup maple syrup

1 tbsp apple cider vinegar 1 tsp vanilla extract

1½ cups whole-wheat flour

½ teaspoon ground cinnamon

½ teaspoon baking soda

¼ cup walnut pieces (optional)

Directions:

1.   Heat the oven to 200°.

2.   Mash the bananas until they reach a puréed consistency (small bits of banana are acceptable). Stir in the vanilla.

3.   Stir in the flour, cinnamon, and baking soda. Fold in the walnut pieces (if using).

4.   Bake for 1 hour, or until you can stick a knife into the middle and it comes out clean.

5.   Let it rest before serving.

Nutritions Per Serving (⅛ loaf):

calories: 178 | fat: 1g | carbs: 40g | protein: 4g | fiber: 5g

Chocolate Pancakes

Preparation Time: 15 minutes

Cooking Time: 30 minutes

Servings: 12

Ingredients:

1¼ cups whole-grain flour 1 tablespoon baking powder

1 tablespoon ground flaxseed

1 tablespoon mini chocolate chips, vegan 2 tablespoons cocoa powder, unsweetened

¼ teaspoon of sea salt

1 tablespoon maple syrup

1 tablespoon apple cider vinegar

1 teaspoon vanilla extract, unsweetened

¼ cup applesauce 1 cup almond milk

Directions:

1.   Take a medium bowl, place whole-grain flour in it, and then whisk in flaxseed, baking powder, cocoa powder, salt, and chocolate chips until well combined.

2.   Take a small bowl, add vinegar, maple syrup, vanilla, and almond milk and whisk until combined.

3.   Whisk well the milk mixture until incorporated, and then let the batter stand for 10 minutes until thickened and doubled in size.

4.   Pour in a saucepan one-twelfth of the batter into the pan, spread it gently; pour in more batter if there is a space on the pan.

5.   Flip the pancake, continue cooking for 2 minutes, and when done, transfer the pancake to a plate.

6.   Serve straight away.

Nutrition:

251.5 Cal 1 g Fat 0.3 g Saturated Fat 58.7 g Carbohydrates 3 g Fiber 5.7 g Sugars; 7 g Protein

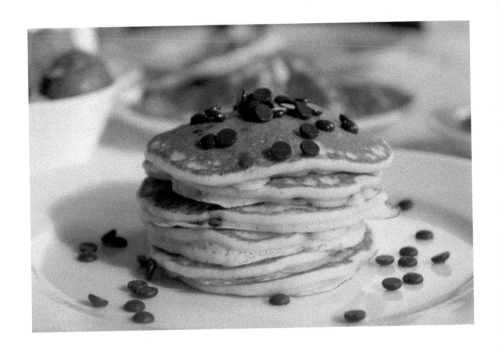

Blueberry and Lemon French Toast

Preparation Time: 15 minutes

Cooking Time: 30 minutes

Servings: 4

Ingredients:

2 tbsp flaxseed 1 tsp ground cinnamon 1/8 tsp sea salt

1/2 teaspoon ground nutmeg 1/2 of a lemon, zested, juiced 2 tablespoons maple syrup

1 teaspoon vanilla extract, unsweetened 1 cup soymilk

1/4 cup hot water

1 cup frozen blueberries

8 slices of whole-grain bread

Directions:

1.   Take a medium bowl, add flaxseeds in it, pour in hot water, stir until just mixed.

2.   Then add salt, all the spices, and vanilla extract, whisk until combined, and whisk in soymilk until incorporated.

3.   Place a large frying pan low heat, spray with oil and wait until hot.

4.   Then soak each bread slice into prepared batter, place it into the frying pan and cook until crispy and nicely brown on all sides; add more soaked slices if there is a space in the pan.

5.   While toasts are being cooked, prepared blueberry syrup, and for this, place a medium heatproof bowl, add blueberries in it, lemon juice and zest, and maple syrup, stir until mixed, and then microwave for 2 minutes until softened.

6.   Serve toasts with prepared blueberry syrup.

Nutrition:

530 Cal 9 g Fat 0.5 g Saturated Fat 92 g Carbohydrates 19 g Fiber 23 g Sugars 21 g Protein

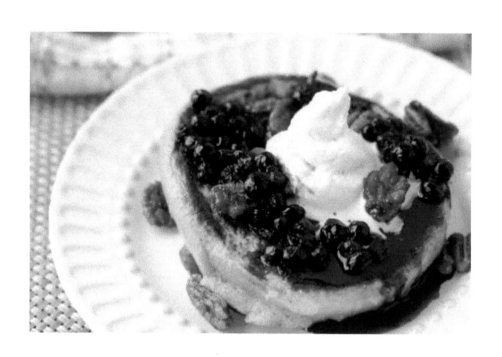

Dairy-Free Coconut Yogurt

Preparation Time: 5 minutes

Cooking Time: 10 minutes

Servings: 2 servings

Ingredients:

1 can coconut milk

4 vegan probiotic capsules

Directions:

1. Shake coconut milk with a whole tube.

2. Remove the plastic of capsules and mix in.

3. Cut a 12-inch cheesecloth until stirred.

4. Freeze or eat immediately.

Nutrition:

Calories: 219 Fat: 10.1g Carbs: 1.5g Protein: 7.9g

Carrot Cake Oats

Preparation time: 6 hours and 10 minutes

Cooking Time: 0 minutes

Servings: 4

Ingredients:

¼ cup shredded carrot 1/3 cup rolled oats

2 tablespoons chopped pineapple

1 tablespoon shredded coconut, unsweetened and more for topping

1 tablespoon ground flaxseed

1 tablespoon raisins and more for topping

2 tablespoons maple syrup and more for topping 1/8 teaspoon ground nutmeg

¼ teaspoon ground cinnamon and more for topping

¼ teaspoon vanilla extract, unsweetened

1 tablespoon chopped walnuts and more for topping

½ cup almond milk, unsweetened

Directions:

1.   Put the ingredients in a bowl and stir until well mixed.

2.   Place the bowl in the refrigerator for a minimum of 6 hours.

3.   When ready to eat, distribute oats mixture evenly among 4 bowls, top with some shredded coconut, raisins, and walnuts, sprinkle with cinnamon, drizzle with maple syrup and then serve.

Nutrition:

Calories: 242 Fat: 9g Carbs: 35g Sugars: 12g Protein: 7g

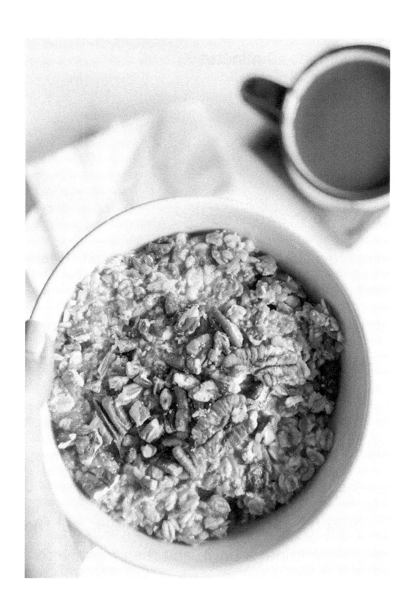

Toast with Avocado and Berries

Preparation Time: 10 minutes

Cooking Time: 10 minutes

Servings: 4

Ingredients:

1 cup sliced strawberries

2 large avocados, peeled, pitted, sliced 4 tablespoons honey

4 slices of whole-grain bread

4oz. block of vegan cheddar cheese, thinly sliced

Directions:

1.   Heat bread slices for 2 to 3 minutes until toasted.

2.   Peel the avocados, remove the pit, cut the flesh in slices, place it into a bowl, and then mash with a fork.

3.   Garnish the toasted slices with avocado, then top with berries and cover with cheese slices.

4.   Drizzle with honey and then serve.

Nutrition:

Calories: 379 Fat: 21g Carbs: 35g Sugars: 9g Protein: 18g

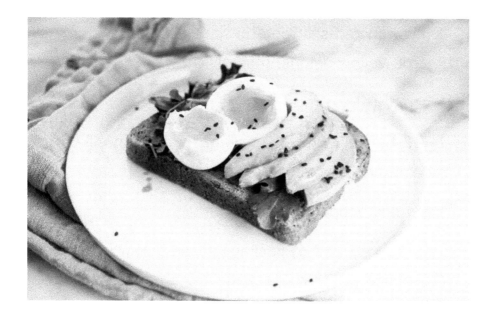

Hearty Breakfast Casserole

Preparation time: 15 minutes

Cook time: 1¼ hours

Serves 6 to 8

Ingredients:

4 medium red-skin potatoes, scrubbed and thinly sliced
3 large yellow onions, thinly sliced

1 pound (454 g) firm tofu

1 (12-ounce / 340-g) package extra-firm silken tofu 2 medium yellow onions, diced

1 red bell pepper, diced

1 (8-ounce / 227-g) package sliced button mushrooms 1 (10-ounce / 283-g) package frozen broccoli, thawed 4 cloves garlic, minced

1 tbsp basil 1 tsp sage

½ teaspoon ground fennel seeds

1 teaspoon crushed red pepper 6 tablespoons nutritional yeast Sea salt, to taste

½ teaspoon black pepper

Directions

1.   Preheat the oven to 350ºF (180ºC).

2.   Steam the potatoes for 6 to 8 minutes, until tender but still firm. While the potatoes steam, sauté the three large onions in a medium skillet until caramelized, about 12 minutes. Set them aside. Place the firm tofu and silken tofu in a large bowl and mash to the consistency of ricotta cheese. Set it aside.

3.   Sautè diced medium onions, red bell peppers, mushrooms, and broccoli for 5 to 6 minutes, until the vegetables are tender. Add the garlic, basil, sage, fennel, and crushed red pepper, and cook for another minute. Add the onion mixture to the tofu along with the nutritional yeast, salt, and pepper. Mix well.

4.   Press the tofu filling into a 9 × 13-inch nonstick baking dish. Top with the steamed potatoes and then the caramelized onions. Bake for 45 minutes.

Southwest Sweet Potato and Mushroom Skillet

Preparation time: 5 minutes

Cook time: 15 minutes

Serves 4

Ingredients:

4 medium sweet potatoes, cut into ½-inch dice 8 ounces (227 g) mushrooms, sliced

1 bell pepper, diced 1 sweet onion, diced

1 cup vegetable broth or water, plus 1 to 2 tablespoons more if needed 1 teaspoon garlic powder

½ teaspoon ground cumin

½ teaspoon chili powder

⅛ teaspoon freshly ground black pepper

Directions:

1.   On medium-low heat put a skillet.

2.   When the skillet is hot, put the sweet potatoes, mushrooms, bell pepper, onion, broth, garlic powder,

cumin, chili powder, and pepper in it and stir. Cover and cook for 10 minutes, or until the sweet potatoes are easily pierced with a fork.

3. Uncover, and give the mixture a good stir. (If any of the contents are beginning to stick to the bottom of the pan, add 1 to 2 tablespoons of broth.)

4. Cook, uncovered, for an additional 5 minutes, stirring once after about 2½ minutes, and serve.

Per Serving

calories: 158 | fat: 1g | carbs: 34g | protein: 6g | fiber: 6g

Strawberry Lemon Protein Muffins

Preparation time: 10 minutes

Cook time: 25 minutes

Serves 6

Ingredients:

2 tbsp chia seeds 5 tbsp butter

½ cup coconut sugar

½ cup plus 2 tbps milk 1 tbsp lemon juice

1½ cups flour

1½ tsp baking powder

½ tsp baking soda

¼ tsp salt

¼ cup raw shelled hemp seeds

½ cup strawberries

Directions:

1.   Let the oven reach 375ºF (190ºC).

2. Grease the inside of a six-cup muffin tin and set aside.

3. Mix 1 tablespoon ground chia seeds together with 3 tablespoons water and set aside.

4. Blend all the ingredients in a mixer. Add the milk and lemon juice. Mix well.

5. Add the flour, baking powder, baking soda, salt, hemp seeds. Combine the mixture with the wet flour. It will be a sticky batter. Fold in the strawberries.

6. Fill at least three-quarters full, even if you're short on filling for one cup. Bake for 25 minutes-

Vegan Green Avocado Smoothie

Preparation Time: 5 minutes

Cooking Time: 10 minutes

Servings: 2 servings

Ingredients:

1 banana

1 cup water 1/2 avocado

1/2 lemon juice

1/2 cup coconut yogurt

Directions:

1. Blend all ingredients until smooth.

Nutrition:

Calories: 299 Fat: 1.1g Carbs: 1.5g Protein: 7.9g

Sun-Butter Baked Oatmeal Cups

Preparation Time: 12 minutes

Cooking Time: 40 minutes

Servings: 12 cups

Ingredients:

1/4 cup coconut sugar 11/2 rolled oats

2 tbsp chia seeds 1/4 teaspoon salt

1   teaspoon cinnamon 1/2 cup non-dairy milk 1/2 cup Sun-Butter

1/2 cup apple sauce

Directions:

1.   preheat oven to 350°F.

2.   Mix all ingredients and blend well.

3.   Add in muffins and insert extra toppings.

4.   Bake 25 minutes, or until golden brown.

Nutrition:

Calories: 129 Fat: 1.1g Carbs: 1.5g Protein: 4.9g

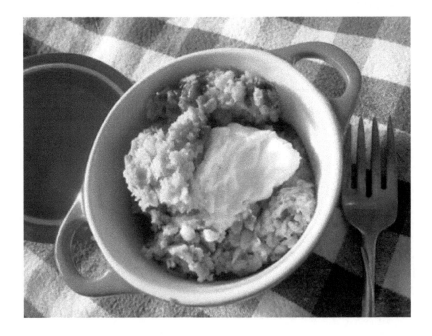

Delicious Quiche made with Cauliflower & Chickpea

Total time: 45 minutes

Ingredients:

½ teaspoon of salt

1 cup of grated cauliflower 1 cup of chickpea flour

½ teaspoon of baking powder

½ zucchini, thinly sliced into half-moons 1 tablespoon of flax meal

1 cup of water

1 freshly chopped sprig of fresh rosemary

½ teaspoon of Italian seasoning

½ freshly sliced red onion

¼ teaspoon of baking powder

Directions

1.   Put together the dry ingredients in a bowl.

2.   Chop the onion and zucchini.

3.   Grate the cauliflower to have a rice-like consistency, and add it to the dry ingredients. Now, add the water and mix well.

4.   Add the zucchini, onion, and rosemary last. You will have a clumpy and thick mixture, but you should be able to spoon it into a tin.

5.   You can use either a silicone or a metal cake tin with a removable bottom. Now put the mixture in the tin and press it down gently.

6.   The top should be left messy to resemble a rough texture.

7.   Bake at $350°$ F for about half an hour. You will know your quiche is ready when the top is golden.

8.   Serve and enjoy!

Tasty Oatmeal and Carrot Cake

Total time: 20 minutes

Ingredients:

1 cup of water

½ teaspoon of cinnamon 1 cup of rolled oats

Salt

¼ cup of raisins

½ cup of shredded carrots 1 cup of non-dairy milk

¼ teaspoon of allspice

½ teaspoon of vanilla extract

Toppings:

¼ cup of chopped walnuts

2 tablespoons of maple syrup

2 tablespoons of shredded coconut

Directions

1.   Bring the non-dairy milk, oats, and water to a simmer.

2.   Now, add the carrots, vanilla extract, raisins, salt, cinnamon, and allspice. You need to simmer all of the ingredients, but do not forget to stir them. You will know that they are ready when the

The liquid is fully absorbed into all of the ingredients (in about 7-10 minutes).

3.   Transfer the thickened dish to bowls.

4.   This nutritious bowl will allow you to kickstart your day.

Go-Green Smoothie

Total time: 10 minutes

Ingredients

2 tablespoons of natural cashew butter 1 ripe frozen banana

2/3 cup of unsweetened coconut, soy, or almond milk 1 large handful of kale or spinach

Directions

1.   Put everything inside a powerful blender.

2.   Blend until creamy.

3.   Enjoy your particular green smoothie.

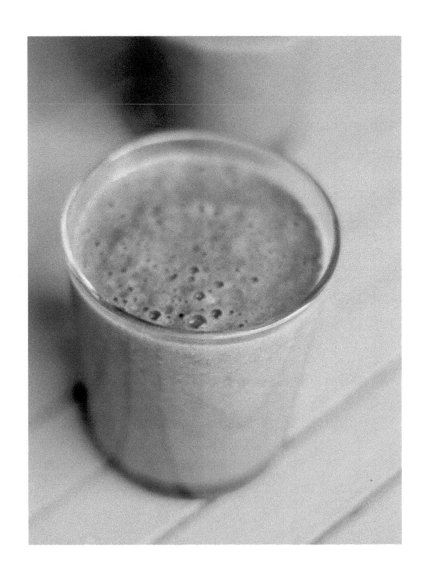

Tasty Oatmeal Muffins

Total time: 30 minutes

Ingredients

½ cup of hot water

½ cup of raisins

¼ cup of ground flaxseed 2 cups of rolled oats

¼ teaspoon of sea salt

½ cup of walnuts

¼ teaspoon of baking soda 1 banana

2 tablespoons of cinnamon

¼ cup of maple syrup

Directions

1.   Whisk the flaxseed with water and allow the mixture to sit for about 5 minutes.

2.   Blend everything for 30 seconds, but do not create a smooth substance. To create rough-textured cookies, you need to have a semi-coarse batter.

3.   Put the batter in cupcake liners and place them in a muffin tin. As this is an oil-free recipe, you will need cupcake liners. Bake everything for about 20 minutes at 350 degrees.

4.   Enjoy the freshly-made cookies with a glass of warm milk.

Sun-Butter Baked Oatmeal Cups

Preparation Time: 10 minutes

Cooking Time: 35 minutes

Servings: 12 cups

Ingredients:

1/4 cup coconut sugar 11/2 rolled oats

2 tbsp chia seeds 1/4 tsp salt

1 teaspoon cinnamon 1/2 cup non-dairy milk 1/2 cup Sun-Butter

1/2 cup apple sauce

Directions:

1.   preheat oven to 350°F.

2.   Mix all Ingredients: and blend well.

3.   Add in muffins and Insert extra toppings.

4.   Bake 25 minutes, or until golden brown.

Nutrition: Calories: 129 Fat: 1.1g Carbohydrates: 1.5g
Protein: 4.9g

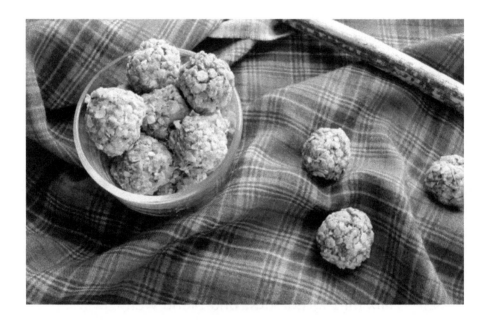

Chocolate Peanut Butter Shake

Preparation Time: 5 minutes

Cooking Time: 5 minutes

Servings: 2 servings

Ingredients:

2 bananas

3 Tablespoons peanut butter 1 cup almond milk

3 Tablespoons cacao powder

Directions:

1. Combine Ingredients: in a blender until smooth.

Nutrition: Calories: 149 Fat: 1.1g Carbohydrates: 1.5g
Protein: 7.9g

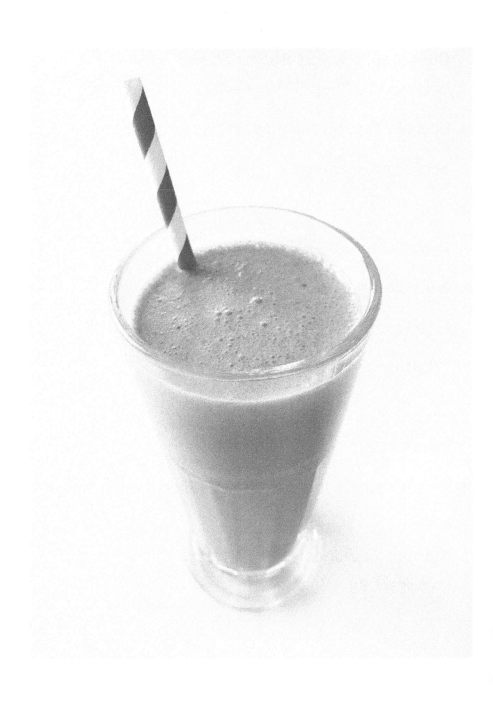

Berries and Banana Smoothie Bowl

Preparation Time: 5 minutes

Cooking Time: 0 minutes

Servings: 4

Ingredients:

For the Smoothie:

4 cups frozen mixed berries 4 small frozen banana, sliced

4 scoops of vanilla protein powder

12 tablespoons almond milk, unsweetened

For the Toppings:

4 tablespoons chia seeds

4 tablespoons shredded coconut, unsweetened 4 tablespoons hemp seeds

½ cup Granola

Fresh strawberries, sliced, as needed

Directions:

1.   Add mixed berries into a food processor along with banana and then pulse at low speed for 1 to 2 minutes until broken.

2.   Add remaining ingredients for the smoothie and then pulse again for 1 minute at low speed until creamy, scraping the sides of the container frequently.

3.   Distribute the smoothie among four bowls, then top with chia seeds, coconut, hemp seeds, granola, and strawberries and serve.

Nutrition: 214 Cal 2.5 g Fat 1.6 g Saturated Fat

47.5 g Carbohydrates 8.8 g Fiber 26 g Sugars 2.8 g Protein;

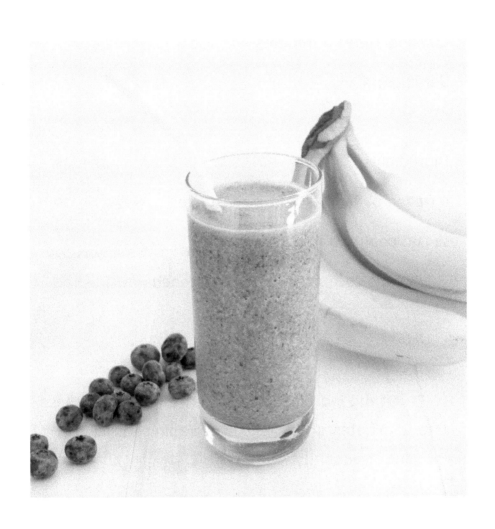

Kale and Peanut Butter Smoothie

Preparation Time: 5 minutes

Cooking Time: 0 minutes

Servings: 4

Ingredients:

4 frozen banana, sliced 2 cups kale

½ cup peanut butter

2 2/3 cups coconut milk, unsweetened

Directions:

1.   Put the ingredients in a blender and then pulse for 1 to 2 minutes until blended, scraping the sides of the container frequently.

2.   Distribute the smoothie among glasses and then serve.

Nutrition: 390 Cal 19 g Fat 2.5 g Saturated Fat 42 g Carbohydrates 7 g Fiber 22 g Sugars 15 g Protein

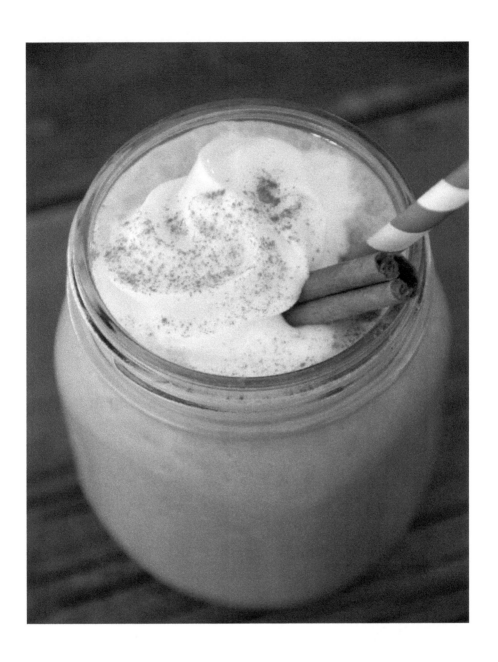

Mint Chocolate Protein Smoothie

Preparation Time: 5 minutes

Cooking Time: 0 minutes

Servings: 4

Ingredients:

4 tablespoons ground flaxseed 4 cups fresh spinach

4 frozen banana, sliced

4 scoops of chocolate protein powder

4 tablespoons chopped dark chocolate, vegan

½ cup melted dark chocolate

1 teaspoon peppermint extract, unsweetened 4 tablespoons honey

3 cups almond milk, unsweetened 1 cup ice cube

Directions:

1.   Put the ingredients in a blender and then pulse for 1 to 2 minutes until blended, scraping the sides of the container frequently.

2.   Distribute the smoothie among glasses and then serve.

Nutrition: 480.5 Cal 20.3 g Fat 8.4 g Saturated Fat 45.6 g Carbohydrates 9.7 g Fiber 22.5 g Sugars 31.2 g Protein;

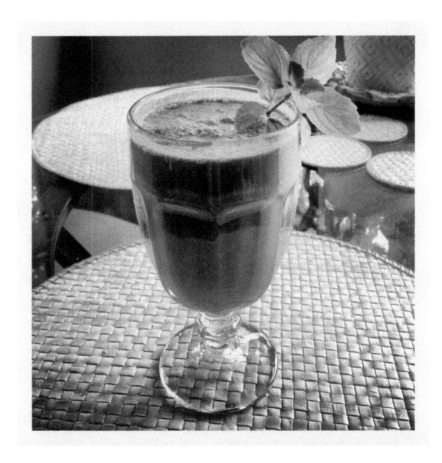

Berry Breakfast Smoothie

Preparation Time: 5 minutes

Cooking Time: 0 minutes

Servings: 4

Ingredients:

2 cups of frozen berries 1 cup oats

1 frozen banana

2 cups vanilla almond milk, unsweetened

Directions:

1.   Put the ingredients in a blender and then pulse for 1 to 2 minutes until blended, scraping the sides of the container frequently.

2.   Distribute the smoothie among glasses and then serve.

Nutrition: 138.5 Cal 2.5 g Fat 0.3 g Saturated Fat 25.6 g Carbohydrates 3.6 g Fiber 6.6 g Sugars 3.5 g Protein

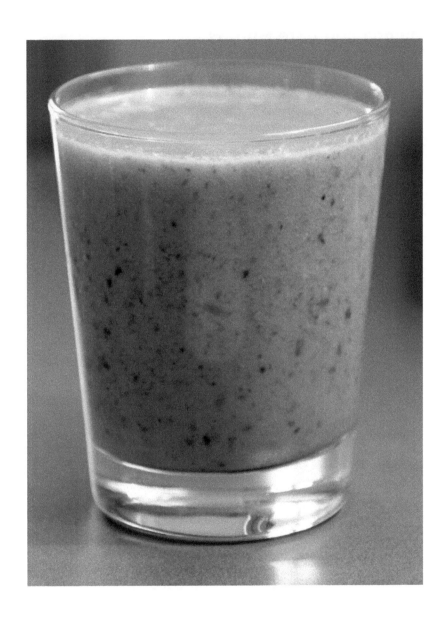

Quinoa and Date Muffins

Preparation time: 10 minutes

Cook time: 40 minutes

Serves 6

Ingredients:

½ cup quinoa

2 tbsp chia seeds

¼ cup almond flour

3 tablespoons vanilla protein powder

½ teaspoon salt

½ cup dates, chopped small 2 tablespoons coconut oil

3 tablespoons maple syrup

1 teaspoon vanilla extract

¼ cup unsweetened shredded coconut

½ cup raisins

Directions:

1.   Cover the quinoa with ½ cup water and bring to a boil over medium-high heat. Cover and turn down to low. Let cook for 20 minutes and then remove from the heat. Take off the lid and let cool.

2.   Turn on the oven to 450ºF (235ºC). Line six muffin cups with paper liners.

3.   Mix the ground chia seeds with ¼ cup plus 2 tablespoons water and set aside.

4.   Add the almond flour, protein powder, and salt to a small bowl. Mix well. Add the dates and mix to coat. Set aside.

5.   Put the coconut oil in a medium bowl. If it is not liquid already, put in the microwave and heat for 10 to 20 seconds or until melted. Remove from microwave and add the maple syrup. Stir well. When cool, add the chia seed mixture, vanilla extract, coconut, almond flour mixture, cooked quinoa, and raisins. Mix well.

6.   Divide the batter between the six muffin cups and bake 12 to 15 minutes, until a toothpick inserted in the center comes out clean.

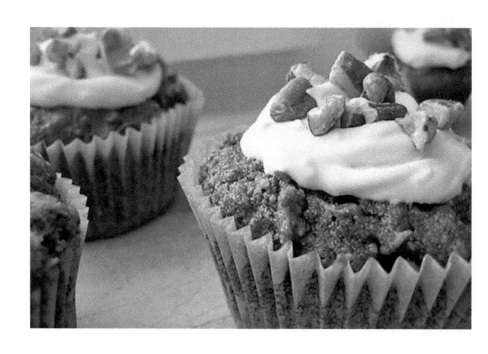

Granola with Nuts and Seeds

Preparation time: 5 minutes

Cook time: 40 minutes

Serves 8

Ingredients:

7 cups old-fashioned oats (use gluten-free if desired) 1 cup shredded coconut

1 cup sunflower seed kernels 1 cup walnuts

1   cup coconut sugar

¼ cup chia (seeds) 1 cup coconut oil 2 cups raisins

Directions:

1.   Preheat the oven to 300ºF (150ºC).

2.   Mix all the ingredients together except for the raisins. Spread out in a large baking pan.

3.   Bake for 40 minutes. Take out of the oven every 10 minutes and stir. Return to the oven.

4.   After 30 minutes, add raisins and stir. Bake for 10 more minutes. Take it out the oven.

5.   Pack in airtight container. Will keep for 4 weeks.

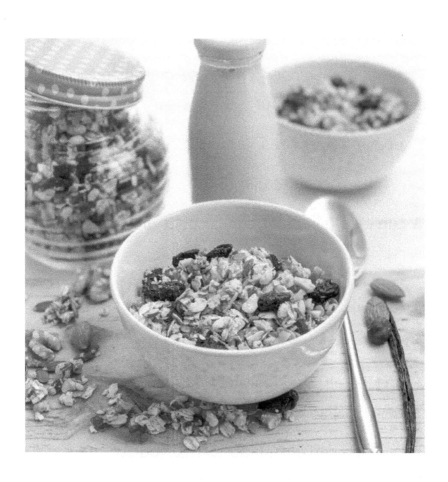

Chocolate Chip and Coconut Pancakes

Preparation Time: 10 minutes

Cooking Time: 40 minutes

Servings: 8

Ingredients:

1¼ cups buckwheat flour

1 tablespoon flaxseeds

2 tablespoons coconut flakes, unsweetened

¼ cup rolled oats 1/8 teaspoon sea salt

1 tablespoon baking powder

1/3 cup mini chocolate chips, vegan

¼ cup maple syrup

1 teaspoon vanilla extract, unsweetened

½ cup applesauce 2 cups almond milk

½ cup of water

bananas, peeled, sliced

Directions:

1.   Put the flaxseeds in a saucepan, pour in water, and then cook for 4 to 5 minutes until sticky mixture comes together.

2.   Strain the flaxseeds mixture immediately into a cup, discard the seeds, and set aside the collected flax water until required.

3.   Take a large bowl, add buckwheat flour and oats in it, and then stir in salt, baking powder, and coconut until mixed.

4.   Take a medium bowl, add 2 tablespoons of reserved flax water along with maple syrup and vanilla, pour in applesauce and milk, and whisk until combined.

5.   Whisk well the milk mixture until thick batter comes together, and fold in chocolate chips.

6.   Take a griddle pan, place it over medium-low heat, spray it with oil and when hot, pour in 1/3 cup of the prepared batter, spread it gently and cook for 5 to 7 minutes until the bottom turns golden brown; pour in more batter if there is a space on the pan.

7.   Flip the pancake, continue cooking for 5 minutes, and when done, transfer pancake to a plate and then repeat with the remaining batter.

8.   Serve pancakes with sliced bananas.

Nutrition:

Calories: 190 Fat: 14g Carbs: 8g Sugars: 18.2g Protein: 8g

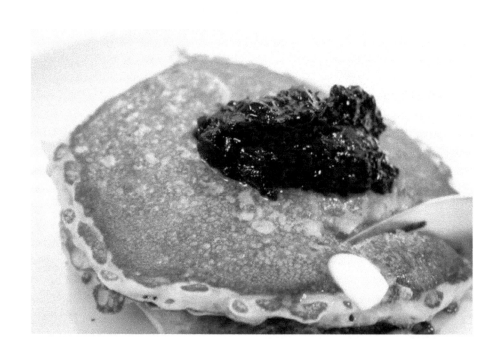

Vegan Blueberry Flax Muffins

Cook Time: 50 minutes

Servings: 12

Ingredients:

1/4 cup ground flax 2 cups oat flour

2 teaspoons baking powder 1 teaspoon vanilla extract

4 tablespoons coconut oil, melted 1 teaspoon vinegar

1 cup almond milk 1/2 cup brown sugar 1/2 cup applesauce

1 1/2 cups blueberries 1/3 cup maple syrup 1/4 teaspoon salt

Instructions:

1.   Preheat the oven to 375 F.

2.   Mix vinegar and almond milk in a bowl and let rest for 10 minutes. Mix flaxseed, flour, salt, baking powder, and cinnamon in a bowl and combine well.

3.   Add coconut oil, applesauce, sugar and almond milk, and vinegar mixture to the flour. Mix gently and fold in the blueberries.

4.   Grease a muffin tray. Fill each of 12 tins with 3/4 way with batter. Bake for 30 minutes. Serve and enjoy.